VETERINARY MANUAL
(WAR) 1915.

FireStep Publishing
Gemini House
136-140 Old Shoreham Road
Brighton
BN3 7BD

www.firesteppublishing.com

First published by the General Staff, War Office 1915.
First published in this format by FireStep Editions,
an imprint of FireStep Publishing, in association with
the National Army Museum, 2013.

www.nam.ac.uk

ISBN 978-1-908487-68-1

Cover design FireStep Publishing
Typeset by FireStep Publishing
Printed and bound in Great Britain

Please note: *In producing in facsimile from original historical documents, any
imperfections may be reproduced and the quality may be lower than modern
typesetting or cartographic standards.*

OFFICIAL COPY

VETERINARY MANUAL (WAR) 1915.

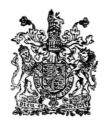

LONDON:
PRINTED UNDER THE AUTHORITY OF HIS MAJESTY'S STATIONERY OFFICE
BY HARRISON AND SONS, ST. MARTIN'S LANE,
PRINTERS IN ORDINARY TO HIS MAJESTY.

FIRESTEP
Editions

www.firesteppublishing.com

MILITARY BOOKS

Published by

Authority.

LONDON:

PRINTED UNDER THE AUTHORITY OF HIS MAJESTY'S STATIONERY OFFICE
By HARRISON AND SONS, 45-47, ST. MARTIN'S LANE, W.C.
PRINTERS IN ORDINARY TO HIS MAJESTY.

To be purchased, either directly or through any Bookseller, from
WYMAN AND SONS, LTD., 29, BREAMS BUILDINGS, FETTER LANE, E.C., and
54, ST. MARY STREET, CARDIFF; or
H.M. STATIONERY OFFICE (SCOTTISH BRANCH), 23, FORTH STREET, EDINBURGH; or
E. PONSONBY, LTD., 116, GRAFTON STREET, DUBLIN;
or from the Agencies in the British Colonies and Dependencies,
the United States of America and other Foreign Countries of
T. FISHER UNWIN, LONDON, W.C

(The prices in brackets are those at which the books are obtainable,
post free, by Officers, Non-Commissioned Officers, and Men, in
the manner prescribed by Appendix XXIII. of The King's
Regulations and Orders for the Army, 1912. Applications
should be made on Army Form L 1372, and addressed to the
Secretary, War Office, S.W.)

ABYSSINIA. Expedition to. 2 vols. and maps. 1870. Half Mor., £5 5s.
Cloth. £4 4s.

AFRICA. Continent of. Geology of. Notes on. 1906. 8s. (2s. 4d.)

AMHARIC LANGUAGE. Short Manual of the. With Vocabulary. 1909. 5s.
(3s. 6d.)

ANIMAL MANAGEMENT. 1908. 1s. 6d. (1s. 4d.)

ARABIC GRAMMAR. Two parts. 1887. (Sold to Officers only) 10s.
(10s. 6d.)

ARMOURERS, Instructions for, in the care, repair, browning, &c., of Small
Arms, Machine Guns, "Parapet" Carriages, and for the care of Bicycles. 1912.
1s. 6d. (1s. 4d.)
Ditto. Amendments. Aug. 1912; Aug. 1914. Each 1d. (1d.)

ARMY ACCOUNTS. (Reprinted from THE ARMY REVIEW, January, 1914.)
3d. (3d.)

ARMY CIRCULARS AND ARMY ORDERS issued before Dec. 31,
1892, which are still in force and required for reference. Reprint of
May, 1896. 3d. (3d.)

ARMY ORDERS. Monthly. Each 8d. (3d.)

ARMY ORDERS. Covers for. 9d. (9d.)

ARMY ENTRANCE Regulations:—
R.M. Academy. Admission to, from April 1, 1912. 1d. (1d.) (Under revision)
R.M. College. Ditto. 1d. (1d.) (Under revision)
Militia and Imperial Yeomanry. Officers of. 1907. 1d. (1d.)
Special Reserve of Officers, Malta Militia, Bermuda Militia, Channel Islands
Militia, and Territorial Force. Officers of the. 1912. 1d. (1d.)
University Candidates. 1912. 1d. (1d.)
Military Forces of the Self-governing Dominions and Crown Colonies.
Officers of the. 1912. 1d. (1d.)
Warrant Officers and N.C.O. of the Regular Army. Combatant Com-
missions as Second Lieutenants. 1914. Provisional. 1d. (1d.)
See also Commission; Medical Corps; Special Reserve; Territorial Force,
Veterinary Corps.

(B 11157) Wt. 1971—707 10M 5/15 H & S

(As to prices in brackets, see top of page 2.)

ARMY LIST. The Quarterly (*not issued in* October, 1914). Each 15*s.* (10*s.* 9*d.*)

ARMY LIST. Monthly. Each 1*s. 6d.* (1*s. 5d.*) (*Not issued in* September, 1914.)

PROMOTIONS, APPOINTMENTS, &c., during August, 1914. [Printed in consequence of the temporary suspension of the Monthly Army List.] 6*d.* (6*d.*)

Ditto, during September 1914. [Ditto.] 6*d.* (7*d.*)

ARMY PAY, Appointment, Promotion, and Non-Effective Pay. Royal Warrant. 1914. 6*d.* (7*d.*)

ARMY ALLOWANCES Regulations. 1914. 6*d.* (6*d.*)

ARMY REVIEW Quarterly. July 1911 to Oct. 1914. 1*s.* (Up to July 1914, 1*s.*; Oct. 1914, 11*d.*) (*Publication suspended.*)

ARMY SERVICE CORPS:—

    Regimental Standing Orders. 1911. 6*d.* (6*d.*); Amendments. 1*d.* (1*d.*)

        Memorandum No. 25. 1*d.* (1*d.*)

    Training. Part I. (Reprinted, with Amendments, 1914). 9*d.* (8*d.*)

                                              (*In the press*)

    Ditto. Part II. Supplies. 1909. (Reprinted, 1914, with new Appendix XII.) 1*s. 3d.* (1*s. 1d.*)

    Ditto. Part III. Transport. 9*d.* (9*d.*)

    Ditto. Part IV. Mechanical Transport. (*Out of print*).

    Ditto. Amendments, July 1914, to Parts I. and III. 3*d.* (3*d.*)

ARTIFICERS. Military. Handbook. 9th edition. 1910. 1*s.* (11*d.*)

                                             (*Under revision*)

Ditto. Amendments. 1912; May 1914. Each. 1*d.* (1*d.*)

ARTILLERY AT THE PICARDY MANŒUVRES IN 1910. Translated from the French. 2*s. 6d.* (2*s.*)

ARTILLERY. Royal:—

    Officers' Mess Management. (*See* Ordnance College.)

    Practice. Instructions—

        Garrison. Coast Defences. Seawards. 1914–15. 3*d.* (3*d.*)

        Garrison. Siege and Movable Armament. 1914. 3*d.* (3*d.*)

        Horse, Field, and Heavy. 1914. 6*d.* (5*d.*)

    Standing Orders for—

        Brigade of Mounted Artillery. 1*d.* (1*d.*)

        Lieut.-Colonel's Command, R.G.A. (Coast and Siege). 1*d.* (1*d.*)

    Training—

        Field. 1914. 9*d.* (9*d.*)

        Garrison—

            Vol. I. 1914. 6*d.* (6*d.*)

            Vol. II. (Siege). 1911. (Reprinted, with Amendments, 1914). 9*d.* (8*d.*)

            Vol. III. 1911. (Reprinted, with Amendments, 1914). 1*s.* (11*d.*)

ARTILLERY COLLEGE. Reports upon the 14th to 18th Senior Classes. Each 1*s.* (9*d.*) (*See also* Ordnance College.)

ARTILLERY. FIELD. The Tactics of. (*Von Schell.*) Translated. 1900. 1*s.* (10*d.*)

ARTILLERY INSTRUMENTS. Handbook of. 1914. 1*s. 6d.* (1*s. 4d.*)

ARTILLERY MUSEUM in the Rotunda, Woolwich. Official Catalogue, 1906. (*Sold at the Rotunda. Price* 1*s. 6d.*)

ARTILLERY AND RIFLE RANGES ACT, 1885, and MILITARY LANDS ACT, 1892. Byelaws under:—

    Aldeburgh, 1896 ; Ash (Aldershot Camp), 1887; Finborough, 1901 ; Hythe, 1894 ; Inchkeith Battery, 1896 ; Kinghornness, 1896 ; Landguard, 1887 ; Lydd—Dungeness, 1895; Middlewick. 1890 ; Millbrook, 1888; Orchard Portman, 1896 ; Scarborough, 1902 ; Scraps Gate, 1886; Shoeburyness, 1895; Southwold, 1896 ; Strensall, 1900 ; Wash, 1891; Whitehaven Battery (Cumberland), 1896. Each 1*d.* (1*d.*)

(As to prices in brackets, see top of page 2.)

Artillery and Rifle Ranges Act, &c.—*continued.*
　Purfleet, 1911.　1*s.*　(9*d.*)
　Salisbury Plain, 1900.　4*d.*　(4*d.*)
ARTILLERY STORE ACCOUNTS AND THE SUPERVISION OF
　R.G.A. SUB-DISTRICTS.　Notes on.　1914.　1*s.*　(10*d.*)
ARTILLERY STORE ACCOUNTS AND THE CARE AND
　PRESERVATION OF EQUIPMENT OF ROYAL ARTILLERY,
　HORSE, FIELD, AND HEAVY BATTERIES.　Notes on.　Sept. 1914.
　6*d.*　(5*d.*)
BARRACKS.　Care of.　Instruction in.　1901.　9*d.*　(7*d.*)
BASHFORTH CHRONOGRAPH.　Experiments with, to determine the
　resistance of the air to the motion of projectiles.　Report on.　1870　1*s.*　(9*d.*)
BAYONET FIGHTING.　Instruction with Service Rifle and Bayonet.
　1915.　1*d.*　(1*d.*)
BAYONET FIGHTING FOR COMPETITIONS.　Instruction in.　1*d.* (1*d.*)
BERMUDA MILITIA ARTILLERY.　Regulations, 1914.　9*d.*　(7*d.*)
BICYCLES. Military.　Handbook on.　1911.　(Reprinted, with Amendments,
　1914).　1*d.*　(1*d.*)
BRITISH MINOR EXPEDITIONS, 1746 to 1814.　1884.　2*s. 6d.*
　(1*s.* 11*d.*)
CADET UNITS.　(*See* Territorial Force.)
CAMEL CORPS TRAINING.　Provisional.　1913.　8*d.*　(7*d.*)
CAPE OF GOOD HOPE.　Reconnaissance Survey of the, 1903-1911.
　Report on the.　1*s. 6d.*　(1*s.* 1*d.*)
CAVALERIE.　Translated from the French of Captain Loir.　(*In the press*)
CAVALRY OF THE LINE.　PEACE ORGANIZATION OF THE;
　and Arrangements for Mobilization consequent on the establishment of
　Cavalry Depôts.　(Special A.O., July 19, 1909).　1*d.*　(1*d.*)
CAVALRY SCHOOL, NETHERAVON.　Standing Orders.　1911.　2*d.*　(2*d.*)
CAVALRY TRAINING.　1912.　(Reprinted, with Amendments, 1914.)
　1*s.*　(10*d.*)　　　　　　　　　　　　　　　　　(*In the press*)
CEREMONIAL.　1912.　3*d.*　(4*d.*);　Provisional Amendments, June 1914.
　1*d.* (1*d.*)
CHEMISTRY.　PRACTICAL.　Quantitative and Qualitative.　A Course
　of.　5*s.*　(3*s.* 8*d.*)
CHEMISTS OF THE RESEARCH DEPARTMENT.　Rules and
　Regulations.　1*d.*　(1*d.*)
CHIROPODY Manual.　2*d.*　(2*d.*)
CIVIL EMPLOYMENT FOR EX-SOLDIERS.　Guide to.　1913.　2*d.* (2*d.*)
CIVIL EMPLOYMENT Regulations.　1913.　1*d.*　(1*d.*)
CIVIL POWER.　DUTIES IN AID OF THE　Special A.O., Dec. 17, 1908.
　(Amendments to "King's Regulations," and to "Manual of Military Law ").　1*d.*
　(1*d.*)
CLOTHING AND NECESSARIES (including Materials).　Priced
　Vocabulary of.　1913.　1*s.*　(11*d.*);　Amendments, July, Oct. 1913;　Jan.,
　April, July 1914.　Each 1*d.*　(1*d.*)
CLOTHING Regulations:—
　　Part I.　Regular Forces (excluding the Special Reserve).　1914.　6*d.*　(6*d.*)
　　Part II.　Special Reserve　1914.　3*a.*　(3*d.*)
　　Part III.　Mobilization, Field Service, and Demobilization.　1908.　3*d.*　(3*d.*)
　　Amendments to Parts I., II , and III.　Nov. 1909;　April, Oct. 1910;　March,
　　　April, Sept., Nov. 1911;　Feb., May, July, Sept. 1912;　April, July
　　　1913.　Each 1*d.*　(1*d.*)
COLCHESTER GARRISON.　Standing Orders.　1913.　9*d.*　(7*d.*)
COMMAND.　ALDERSHOT.　Standing Orders.　1914.　2*s. 3a.*　(1*s.* 9*d.*)
COMMAND.　THE ART OF.　By Colonel von Spohn.　Translated.　1*d.*　(1*d.*)
COMMAND.　WESTERN.　Standing Orders.　Jan. 1910.　(Reprinted, with
　Amendments, 1915).　6*d.*　(5*d.*)

(As to prices in brackets, see top of page 2.)

COMMANDS, Military, and Staff in the United Kingdom. Reorganization of. (Special A.O., Jan. 6, 1905, with alterations to date. Issued with Special A.O., Nov. 11, 1907.) 3*d.* (3*d.*)

COMMISSION IN H.M. REGULAR ARMY (from 1st April, 1912). Short guide to the various ways of obtaining a; &c., &c. April 1912. 2*d.* (2*d.*) (*See also* Army Entrance; Medical Corps; Special Reserve; Territorial Force; Veterinary Corps.)

COMPANY TRAINING. Notes on. For the use of the Special Reserve, Territorial Force, and newly-raised Units of the Regular Army. Sept. 1914. 1*d.* (1*d.*)

CONVEYANCE OF TROOPS AND ISSUE OF TRAVELLING WARRANTS. Instructions. 1910. 2*d.* (2*d.*)

COOKING. Military. Manual of. 6*d.* (5*d.*)

COOKING AND DIETARY. Military. Manual of. 1915. Mobilization. 2*d.* (2*d.*)

COURSES OF INSTRUCTION, 1914–15. 2*d.* (2*d.*) Ditto, at Practice Camps, 1914. 1*d.* (1*d.*)

CREWS OF WAR DEPARTMENT VESSELS AND BOATS AT HOME STATIONS. Regulations for the Appointment, Pay, and Promotion of. 1911. 2*d.* (2*d.*)

CYCLIST TRAINING. Provisional. 1914. 3*d.* (3*d.*)

DIVISION ORDERS. Extracts from. 1880. 2*s.* 6*d.* (1*s.* 9*d.*)

DRAINAGE MANUAL. 1907. 2*s.* 6*d.* (2*s.*)

DRAWING PLATES. Military:—
Attack of Dufor's Countermines or 2nd plate of Mines; Carnot's First System; Detached Forts; Concealed Defences, 1, 2, 3, 4; Printing Plate, A, B, C, &c.; Detail Plate, No. 1; Do. No. 2; Neighbourhood of Woolwich; Village and Surrounding Ground. Each 2*d.* (2*d.*)
Attack of Fortress—Preliminary Operations; Do., Distant Attack; Do., Close Attack; Neighbourhood of Metz. Each 3*d.* (3*d.*)
Woods and Villages. 6 plates. Each 6*d.* (5*d.*)
Neighbourhood of Woolwich. Southern Side. 1*s.* 6*d.* (1*s.* 1*d.*)

DRESS REGULATIONS. 1911. 2*s.* 6*d.* (2*s.*); Amendments, March, Aug. 1912. Each 1*d.* (1*d.*); Aug. 1913. 2*d.* (2*d.*)

DRUM AND FLUTE DUTY for the Infantry, with Instructions for the Training of Drummers and Flautists. 1887. 2*s.* (1*s.* 6*d.*)

DYNAMICS. Notes on. (*See* Ordnance College.)

EGYPT. BRITISH FORCE IN. Standing Orders. 1912. 1*s.* (10*d.*)

EGYPT. CAMPAIGN OF 1882 IN. Military History. With case of Maps. Condensed Edition. 1908. 3*s.* 6*d.* (2*s.* 8*d.*)

ELECTRICAL COMMUNICATIONS. FIXED. Instructions as to. 1912. 4*d.* (4*d.*)

ELECTRICITY AND MAGNETISM. Text Book for use of the Cadets at the R.M. Academy. 1911. 2*s.* 6*d.* (2*s.*)

ELECTRICITY. Notes on. 1911. 1*s.* 3*d.* (1*s.* 1*d.*)

ELECTRIC LIGHT APPARATUS. DEFENCE. Instructions for the Working of. 1911. 1*d.* (1*d.*)

ELECTRIC LIGHTING. Military. Vol. I. 1*s.* (11*d.*); Vol. II (Reprinted, with Amendments, 1915). (*In the press*); Vol. III. 1*s.* (11*d.*)

ENCOUNTER. THE BATTLE OF. By Hans von Kiesling. Part I. Practical. Translated. 1*s.* 6*d.* (1*s.* 3*d.*)

ENGINEER SERVICES Regulations. Peace:—Part I. 1910. 1*s.* (10*d.*) Part II. 1911. Technical Treatises. 9*d.* (7*d.*)

ENGINEER TRAINING. 1912. (Reprinted, with Amendments, 1914). 6*d.* (6*d.*)

ENGINEERING. Field. Manual of. 1911. (Reprinted 1913). 9*d.* (9*d.*)

(As to prices in brackets, see top of page 2.)

ENGINEERING. Military :—

Part I. Field Defences. 1908. **1s. 6d.** (1s. 3d.)
Part II. Attack and Defence of Fortresses. 1910. 9d. (8d.)
Part IIIa. Military Bridging.—General Principles and Materials. 1913.
1s. (11d.)
Part IIIb. Ditto.—Bridges. 1913. 3d. (1s. 2d.)
Part IV. Mining and Demolitions. 1910. 1s. (11d.)
Part V. Miscellaneous. 1914. 1s. (11d.)
Part VI. Military Railways. 1898. *(Out of print)*

EQUIPMENT. INFANTRY. Pattern 1908 Web. 1913. 2d. (2d.)

EQUIPMENT Regulations :—

Part 1. 1912. (Reprinted, with Amendments published in Army Orders
up to Aug. 31, 1914). 1s. (11d.)
Part 2. Details—

Sect.
I. Infantry. (Regular Army.) 1913.
6d. (5d.)
Ia. Mounted Infantry. 1912. 6d. (5d.)
II. Cavalry. (Regular Army.) 1914.
3d. (3d.)
III. Army Service Corps. (Regular
Army.) 1913. 6d. (5d.)
IV., IVa., and IVb. Army Ordnance
Corps. Army Pay Corps. Army
Veterinary Corps. (Regular
Army.) 1914. 2d. (2d.)
V. Royal Army Medical Corps. (Regular Army.) 1914. 2d. (2d.)
VI.-IX. R.M. Academy; R.M. and
Staff Colleges ; Garrison Staff
and Schools of Instruction; Military Prisons, Detention Barracks
and Military Provost Staff Corps.
(Regular Army.) 1914. 2d. (2d.)
Xa. Engineer. General. Fortress,
Survey, Railway, and Depôt
Units. Peace and War. (Regular
Army.) 1914. 2d. (2d.)
Xb. Field Troop. (Regular Army.)
1912. 2d. (2d.)
Xc. Field Company. (Regular Army.)
1914. 2d. (2d.)
Xd. Divisional Signal Company. (Regular Army.) 1914. 2d. (2d.)
Xe. Signal Company (Wireless). (Regular Army.) 1912. 2d. (2d.)
Xf. Headquarters Signal Units. (Regular Army.) 1914. 2d. (2d.)
Xg. Signal Company (Cable). (Regular Army.) 1912. 2d. (2d.)
Xh. Signal Squadron. (Regular Army.)
1914. 2d. (2d.)
Xj. Signal Troop with Cavalry Brigade.
(Regular Army.) 1912. 2d. (2d.)
Xk. Signal Troop with a Cavalry Brigade not allotted to a Cavalry
Division. (Regular Army.) 1914.
2d. (2d.)
Xl. Signal Company (South Africa).
(Regular Army.) 1912. 2d. (2d.)
Xm. Bridging Train. (Regular Army.)
1912. 2d. (2d.)

Sect.
Xn. Field Squadron. (Regular Army.)
1914. 2d. (2d.)
XIa. Horse Artillery. Q.F. 13-pr.
1913. 9d. (8d.)
XIb. Field Artillery. Q.F. 18-pr.
(Regular Army.) 1914. 9d. (8d.)
XIc. Field Artillery. Q.F. 4·5-in.
Howitzer. (Regular Army.) 1913.
9d. (8d.)
XId. Reserve Brigades with Q.F. 18-pr.
Equipment. Horse and Field
Artillery, Staff and Depôts,
Riding Establishment, School
of Gunnery (Horse and Field),
and Mounted Band. (Regular
Army.) 1914. 6d. (6d.)
XIe. Mountain Artillery with B.L.
2·75 - inch Equipment. Mountain Battery and Ammunition
Column. Mule Transport. Provisional. (Regular Army.) 1914.
6d. (5d.)
XIIa. Royal Garrison Artillery.
(Regular Army.) 1914. 2s. 6d.
(1s. 11d.)
XIIb. Royal Garrison Artillery, Siege
Artillery, Movable Armament,
and Machine Guns in Armaments. 1913. 1s. (10d.)
XIIc. Heavy Artillery. B.L. 60-pr.
(Regular Army.) 1913. 9d. (8d.)
XIV. Cavalry School, Netheravon.
(Regular Army.) 1914. 2d. (2d.)
XV. Camel Corps School, Egypt.
(Regular Army.) 1914. 2d. (2d.)
XVI. Special Reserve. 1913. 4d. (4d.)
XVII. Officers Training Corps. 1912.
3d. (3d.)

Practice Batteries and Drill Guns (Fixed
Mountings) of the Royal Garrison
Artillery. (Part 2. Sections XIIa
and XVI, and Part 3.) 1909.
1s. 6d. (1s. 2d.)

(As to prices in brackets, see top of page 2.)

Equipment Regulations—*continued.*

> Part 3. Territorial Force. 1914. 6*d.* (6*d.*)
> Ditto. Details:—
>> Sec. IX. Artillery. 1912. 1*s.* (9*d.*)
>> Ditto. Amendments, April 1912: Feb. 1914. Each 1*d.* (1*d.*)
>> Sec. X. Engineer. 1912. 3*d.* (3*d.*)
> Amendments to Part 2. Feb., April, July (two issues). Aug. 1914. Each 1*d.* (1*d.*)
> Amendments to Parts 1, 2, and 3. Nov. 1913. 1*d.* (1*d.*)
> Amendments to Parts 1, 2, and 3. Mar., July 1913: April. Aug. 1914. Each 2*d.* (2*d.*)

ESTABLISHMENTS:—

PEACE :—
> Part II. Territorial Force. 1913–14. 4*d.* (4*d.*)   (*Under revision*)
> Ditto. Changes in. Nov. 1913. 1*d.* (1*d.*)
> Part III. Departmental and Miscellaneous Regular Establishments and Instructional Institutions. 1913–14. 2*d.* (2*d.*)
> Part IV. Headquarters Establishments. Home, Colonies and India. 1913–14. 3*d.* (3*d.*)
> Part V. Establishment of Commands Abroad and Summaries of the Military Forces of the Crown. 1913–14. 2*d.* (2*d.*)

WAR :—
> Part I. Expeditionary Force. 1914. 8*d.* (8*d.*)   (*Under revision*)
> Part II. Territorial Force. 1911. 8*d.* (7*d.*)
> Part V. Reserve, Depôt, and other Regimental Units maintained at Home after Mobilization. 1914. 4*d.* (4*d.*)
> Part VI. Departmental and Miscellaneous Regular Establishments and Instructional Institutions maintained at Home after Mobilization. 1914. 2*d.* (2*d.*)
> New Armies. 1915. 2*d.* 3*d.*

EUROPEAN WAR, 1914–15. Despatches (Naval and Military) relating to Operations in the War. Sept., Oct., and Nov., 1914. With List of Honours and Rewards Conferred. With Sketch Map. 2*d.* (3*d.*)

EXAMINATION PAPERS:—

> **Qualifying Certificates.** Sept. 1905 ; March 1906 ; Sept. 1909 ; March, Sept. 1910 ; March, Sept. 1911 ; March 1912. Each 6*d.* (5*d.*)
> **Entrance:** R.M. Academy, R.M. College, Qualifying Test for Commissions. Supplementary First Appointments in the Royal Marines. June–July 1912. 1*s.* (11*d.*)
> **Entrance :** R.M. Academy, R.M. College, Qualifying Test for Commissions. Nov. 1912; Nov.-Dec. 1913. Each 1*s.* (11*d.*)
> **Entrance :** R.M. Academy, R.M. College, Qualifying Test for Commissions. Supplementary First Appointments in the Royal Marines. Appointments in the Indian Police Force. Appointments in the Police Forces of the Straits Settlements and the Federated Malay States. Cadetships in the Royal Navy (Special Entry). June–July 1914. 1*s.* (11*d.*)
> Entrance: R.M. Academy, R.M. College. Nov.-Dec. 1914. 1*s.* (10*d.*)
> Freehand Drawing at the Army Entrance Examination of Nov. 1913. Specimen Paper to illustrate the kind of questions that will be set in. 6*d.* (5*d.*)
> R.M. Academy, Fourth Class; R.M. College, Fourth, Third, and Second Divisions. July, Dec. 1904; June 1905. Each 1*s.*
> R.M. Academy, Fourth Class; R.M. College, Senior Division. Dec. 1905; June, Dec. 1906 ; July, Dec. 1907. Each 1*s.*

(As to prices in brackets, see top of page 2.)

Examination Papers—*continued.*

Staff College. Admission. Aug. 1907 ; Aug. 1909; July 1911 ; June–July 1912 ; June-July 1913. Each 1*s.* (*6d.*)

Regular Forces. Canadian Permanent Forces, Special Reserve of Officers, Territorial Force, and Colonial Military Forces. May, Nov. 1906; May, Nov. 1908. Each 1*s.* (*11d.*)

Ditto. May 1909. 9*d.* (*8d.*)

Officers for Promotion. Dec. 1912 ; May, Dec. 1913 ; April 1914. Each 1*s.* (*6d.*)

Militia, Imperial Yeomanry, and University Candidates. Mar., Sept. 1904 ; Sept. 1905; Oct. 1906. Each 1*s.*

Special Reserve, Militia, Territorial Force, and University Candidates. Oct. 1911; March, Oct. 1912 ; March, Oct. 1913. Each 1*s.* (*6d.*)

Special Reserve, Military, Territorial Force, Non-Commissioned Officers, and University Candidates. March 1914. 1*s.* (*6d.*)

Officers' Training Corps:—

Cadets of the Senior Division. Certificate A. Dec. 1908. 6*d.* (*5d.*) •

Cadets of the Junior and Senior Divisions. Certificates A and B. Spring of 1909; Nov. 1910 ; May, Nov. 1911 ; March, Nov. 1912 ; March, Nov. 1913 ; March 1914. Each 6*d.* (*6d.*)

Foreign Languages. Modern. July, 1906 ; July 1908; April, July 1909; Jan., June, Oct. 1910 ; Jan., June, Oct. 1911 ; June 1912 ; June 1913 ; June 1914. Each 1*s.* (*6d.*)

EXPLOSIVES. Service. Treatise on. 1907. 1*s.* 6*d.* (1*s.* 2*d.*)

FIELD ALMANAC. 1915. 1*d.* (1*d.*)

FIELD SERVICE. Manual for:—

Artillery. Field. Brigade. Q.F. 18-pr. 1908. 3*d.* (3*d.*) (*Under revision*)

Ditto. Ditto. (Howitzer) Brigade. 5-inch B.L. 1908. 3*d.* (3*d.*)

Ditto. Heavy (B.L. 60-pr.) Battery and Ammunition Column. Expeditionary Force. 1910. 3*d.* (3*d.*)

Ditto. Horse. Brigade. 13-pr. Q.F. 1908. 3*d.* (3*d.*) (*Under revision*)

Ditto. Ditto. Appendix to. R.H.A. Battery and Mounted Brigade Ammunition Column. 1*d.* (1*d.*)

Cavalry Regiment. Expeditionary Force. 1913. 3*d.* (3*d.*) (*Under revision*)

Engineers. Palloon Company. Expeditionary Force. 1910. 3*d.* (3*d.*)

Ditto. Bridging Train. Expeditionary Force. 1915. 3*d.* (3*d.*)

Ditto. Field Company. Expeditionary Force. 1915. 3*d.* (3*d.*)

Ditto. Field Squadron. Expeditionary Force. 1914. 3*d.* (3*d.*)

Ditto. Works Company. Expeditionary Force. 1910. 3*d.* (3*d.*)

Headquarters Units. Expeditionary Force. 1911. 3*d.* (3*d.*)

Infantry Battalion. Expeditionary Force. 1914. 3*d.* (3*d.*)

Infantry (Mounted) Battalion. Expeditionary Force. 1913. 3*d.* (3*d.*)

Medical Service. Army. Expeditionary Force. 1914. 3*d.* (3*d.*)

Signal Service. Signal Company (Air-Line). Expeditionary Force. 1913. 3*d.* (3*d.*)

Ditto. Ditto. (Cable). Expeditionary Force. 1913. 3*d.* (3*d.*)

Ditto. Ditto. (Divisional). Expeditionary Force. 1915 3*d.* (3*d.*)

Ditto. Ditto. (Lines of Communication). Expeditionary Force. 1914. 3*d.* (3*d.*)

FIELD SERVICE POCKET BOOK. 1914. 1*s.* (11*d.*)

(As to prices in brackets, see top of page 2.)

FIELD SERVICE REGULATIONS:—

Part I. Operations. 1909. (Reprinted, with Amendments. 1914). 6d. (6d.)

Part II. Organization and Administration. 1909. (Reprinted, with Amendments to Oct. 1914). 1s. (10d.)

Ditto. Amendments, April 1915. 1d (1d.)

FINANCIAL INSTRUCTIONS IN RELATION TO ARMY ACCOUNTS. 1910. (Reprinted, with Amendments to Sept. 1, 1914). 4d. (4d.)

FLYING CORPS. ROYAL. Training Manual:—

Part I. Provisional. 1914. 1s. (10d.)

Ditto. Amendments. Jan. 1915. 1d. (1d.)

Part II. Military Wing. Provisional. 1914. 3d. (4d.)

FOREIGN LANGUAGES. STUDY OF. Regulations. 1913. 2d. (2d.)

FORTIFICATION. PERMANENT. For the Imperial Military Training Establishments and for the Instruction of Officers of all Arms of the Austro-Hungarian Army. 7th Edition. Translated. 4s. (2s. 11d.)

FRANCO-GERMAN WAR, 1870-71. Translated from the German Official Account. Five Vols. £6 11s. 6d.

Also separately, in Volumes in cloth, Sections in paper covers, and Plans unmounted :—

First Part—History of the War to the Downfall of the Empire—

Vol. 1 (Secns. 1 to 5). Outbreak of Hostilities to Battle of Gravelotte. £1 6s. *(Out of print)*

Vol. 2 (Secns. 6 to 9). Battle of Gravelotte to Downfall of the Empire. £1 2s. *(Out of print)*

Second Part—History of the War against the Republic—

Vol. 1 (Secns. 10 to 13). Investment of Paris to Re-occupation of Orleans by the Germans. £1 6s. (18s. 6d.)

Vol. 2 (Secns. 14 to 18). Events in Northern France from end of Nov. In North-west from beginning of Dec. Siege of Paris from commencement of Dec. to the Armistice. Operations in the south-east from middle of Nov. to middle of Jan. £1 6s. (19s.)

Vol. 3 (Secns. 19 and 20). Events in South-east France from middle of Jan. to Termination of Hostilities. Rearward Communications. The Armistice. Homeward March and Occupation. Retrospect. £1 11s. 6d. (£1 2s. 6d.)

Section.

1. Events in July. Plan. 3s. (2s. 2d.)

2. Events to Eve of Battles of Wörth and Spicheren. 3rd edition. 3s. *(Out of print)*

3. Battles of Wörth and Spicheren. 3rd edition. 5s. *(Out of print)*

4. Advance of Third Army to the Moselle, &c. 2nd edition. 4s. *(Out of print)*

5. Operations near Metz on 15th, 16th, and 17th August. Battle of Vionville—Mars la Tour. 2nd edition. 6s. 6d. *(Out of print)*

6. Battle of Gravelotte—St. Privat. 5s. *(Out of print)*

7. Advance of Third Army and of Army of the Meuse against Army of Chalons. 6s. *(Out of print)*

8. Battle of Sedan. 3s. *(Out of print)*

9. Proceedings on German Coast and before Fortresses in Alsace and Lorraine. Battle of Noisseville. General Review of War up to September. 4s. 6d. (3s. 4d.)

10. Investment of Paris. Capture of Toul and Strassburg. 6s (4s. 6d.)

11. Events before Paris, and at other points of Theatre of War in Western France until end of October. 5s. 3d. (3s. 11d.)

12. Last Engagements with French Army of the Rhine. Occurrences after fall of Strassburg and Metz to middle of November. 4s. 6d. (3s. 5d.)

13. Occurrences on Theatre of War in Central France up to Re-occupation of Orleans by the Germans. 6s. (4s. 6d.)

9

(As to prices in brackets, see top of page 2.)

Franco-German War—*continued.*

Section.

14. Measures for Investment of Paris up to middle of December. **4s.** (*3s.*)
15. Measures for protecting the Investment of Paris and Occurrences before French Capital to commencement of 1871. **2s. 6d.** (*1s. 11d.*)
16. Proceedings of Second Army from commencement of 1871 until the Armistice. **3s. 6d.** (*2s. 8d.*)
17. Proceedings of First Army from commencement of 1871 until the Armistice. **3s.** (*2s. 3d.*)
18. Occurrences on South-eastern Theatre of War up to middle of Jan. 1871. Events before Paris from commencement of 1871 to the Armistice. **8s.** (*6s.*)
19. Occurrences on South-eastern Theatre of War from middle of January, 1871. Proceedings in rear of German Army and in Coast Provinces from Nov., 1870 until the Armistice. **13s. 6d.** (*9s. 8d.*)
20. General Retrospect of War from beginning of Sept., 1870 to Cessation of Hostilities. Armistice and Peace Preliminaries. Return of German Army and Peace of Frankfort. The Occupation. The Telegraph, Post, Supply of Ammunition, Commissariat, Hospital Service, Divine Service, Military Justice, Recruitment, and Home Garrisons. Results. **5r.** (*3s, 9d.*)

Analytical Index. **1s. 6d.** (*1s. 1d.*)

Plans—

4. Battle of Colombey-Nouilly. **3d.** (*3d.*)
5A. Battle of Vionville—Mars la Tour. Position of Contending Forces at Noon. **3d.** (*3d.*)
5B. Battle of Vionville—Mars la Tour. Position of Contending Forces from 4 to 5 p.m. **3d.** (*3d.*)
9A. Battle of Sedan. Position of Contending Forces towards Noon. **3d.** (*3d.*)
9B. Battle of Sedan. Position of the Germans in the afternoon shortly before the end of the struggle. **3d.** (*3d.*)

(*See also* SIEGE OPERATIONS.)

GERMAN ARMY. Cavalry. Drill Regulations. 1909. **3d.** (*3d.*)
Ditto. Field Service Regulations. 1908. **1s.** (*10d.*)
Ditto. Foot Artillery. Drill Regulations. Part IV. THE FIGHT. 1909. **3d.** (*3d.*)
Ditto. Manœuvres Regulations. 1908. **3d.** (*3d.*)

GERMANY. The Campaign of 1866 in. With 22 Plans in portfolio. 1872. (Reprinted 1907). **6s.** (*4s. 10d.*)

Ditto. Moltke's Projects for. **1s.** (*10d.*)

GUERNSEY AND ALDERNEY ROYAL MILITIA. Regulations. With the Militia Laws relating to the Islands. Provisional. **3s.** (*2s. 2d.*)

GUNS. Drill for. (*And see* **GUNS.** Handbooks for):—

60-pr. B.L. (Reprinted, with Amendments 1915). 1912. **1d.** (*1d.*)
(*In the press*)

18-pr. Q.F. 1914. **1d.** (*1d.*)
15-pr. B.L. 1914. **1d.** (*1d.*)
15-pr. B.L.C. 1914. **1d.** (*1d.*)
15-pr. Q.F. 1912. **1d.** (*1d.*)
13-pr. Q.F. 1914. **1d.** (*1d.*)
12-pr. 12-cwt. Q.F. Land Service. 1914. **1d.** (*1d.*)
10-pr. B.L. 1914. **1d.** (*1d.*)
9·2-inch B.L. Mark IX., on Mark IV. Mounting. Land Service. 1914. **1d.** (*1d.*)
9·2-inch B.L. "C" Mark IX., on Marks VA. and VB. Mountings. Land Service. 1914. **1d.** (*1d.*)
9·2-inch B.L. Marks X., Xv., and X*., on Mark V. Mounting. Land Service. 1914. **1d.** (*1d.*)

VETERINARY MANUAL
(WAR), 1915.

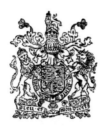

LONDON:
PRINTED UNDER THE AUTHORITY OF HIS MAJESTY'S STATIONERY OFFICE
By HARRISON AND SONS, 45-47, St. Martin's Lane, W.C.,
Printers in Ordinary to His Majesty.

To be purchased, either directly or through any Bookseller, from
WYMAN AND SONS, LTD., 29, BREAMS BUILDINGS, FETTER LANE, E.C., and
54, St. Mary Street, Cardiff; or
H.M. STATIONERY OFFICE (Scottish Branch), 23, Forth Street, Edinburgh; or
E. PONSONBY, LTD., 116, Grafton Street, Dublin;
or from the Agencies in the British Colonies and Dependencies,
the United States of America and other Foreign Countries of
T. FISHER UNWIN, London, W.C.

1915.

Price One Penny.

CONTENTS.

(B 11157) Wt. w. 12231—1584 10m 4/15 H & S P. 15/99

1. ORGANIZATION.

1. The Veterinary Service of an Army in the field is organized and controlled by a Director of Veterinary Services. Its function is to promote efficiency by preventing and reducing wastage amongst the animals of the Army.

2. The general principles governing this service are contained in Field Service Regulations, Part II, and more detailed instructions as to their execution are given in this manual.

3. Veterinary hospitals are located on the Lines of Communication for the treatment and care of sick and injured animals of the field army. Mobile Veterinary Sections are provided to relieve field units of all sick and injured animals, and convey them to veterinary hospitals.

4. Base and advanced veterinary store depots are formed for the upkeep of veterinary equipment.

5. The personnel allotted to the above units is laid down in War Establishments.

2. DIRECTOR OF VETERINARY SERVICES.

1. The duties of the Director of Veterinary Services are defined in Field Service Regulations, Part II, Chapter III.

2. He advises on all technical matters, and subject to the instructions of the Commander-in-Chief (or of I.G.C.), conveyed to him through the Quartermaster-General's branch of the staff, controls all arrangements in connection with the Veterinary Service. He commands and is responsible for the distribution and co-ordinate working of the veterinary personnel with the force. He is assisted by one or more Deputy-Directors, and is represented in divisional commands by Assistant Directors.

3. The offices of the Director and Deputy-Director or Directors will be located as may be ordered from time to time by the Commander-in-Chief.

4. The Director or a Deputy-Director will, when necessary, precede the Army to the theatre of war and make such preparatory veterinary arrangements at the base and Line of Communications as may be necessary for its reception.

5. He will draft such orders as may be necessary in connection with the veterinary arrangements of the force, and will keep such diaries and records of veterinary work in the field as may be required. He communicates directly with his representatives on all matters of technical detail in connection with his service.

6. He will carry out such inspections and make such recommendations as he may consider necessary regarding the health and efficiency of the animals of the force, and will closely supervise the veterinary arrangements.

7. He will take necessary measures to prevent the retention of sick and injured animals not likely to become serviceable again.

8. The duties of the Director with reference to the provision of veterinary stores are referred to in Section 13.

3. DEPUTY-DIRECTORS OF VETERINARY SERVICES.

The duties of a Deputy-Director of Veterinary Services are broadly those indicated for the Director, differing only in degree ; his responsibilities being confined to that portion of the force to which he is accredited.

4. ASSISTANT DIRECTOR OF VETERINARY SERVICES OF A DIVISION.

1. The Assistant Director of Veterinary Services is the responsible adviser of the commander and his staff on all technical matters appertaining to the veterinary service of the division.

2. He administers the personnel of the Army Veterinary Corps allotted to the division, and in regard to technical matters controls and issues orders to them directly. Orders and instructions in respect of other matters affecting the veterinary personnel allotted to units are communicated to commanders of brigades and units.

3. Under the orders of the divisional commander, and in consultation with the staff and representatives of other services concerned, the Assistant Director of Veterinary Services will, when necessary, draft paragraphs regarding veterinary matters for inclusion in divisional orders.

4. He will forward direct to the officer in charge of advanced veterinary store depot all requisitions for veterinary medicines and equipment required by units in the division, duly examining them with a view to the prevention of waste, and the exercise of all possible economy.

5. He will furnish to the Director of Veterinary Services every Sunday, a telegraphic state under the following headings :— " Remaining Last Report," " Admitted Since," " Cured," " Transferred Sick," " Died," " Destroyed," " Missing," " Remaining Under Treatment," and " Total Strength of Formation." This state will include casualties up to and for the previous Thursday, and will be supported by Army Form " A 2000 " rendered by post. A copy of the telegraphic report will be sent for information of the Deputy-Director of Veterinary Services, and a duplicate of the Army Form A 2000 to the Officer i/c Army Veterinary Records at the Base for statistical purposes.

6. In subordinate commands to which no assistant director is allotted, the senior officer, Army Veterinary Corps, is the representative of the Director of Veterinary Services, and the

responsibility for the efficient administration of the veterinary
service in the command will devolve on him. His duties are
analogous to those of an Assistant Director of Veterinary Services,
and will be performed in addition to his executive duties.

5. OFFICERS ATTACHED TO UNITS.

1. A veterinary officer attached to a unit is responsible for the
treatment of all sick and injured animals with that unit. He will
advise commanders of units which animals should be transferred
to mobile sections for conveyance to veterinary hospitals, and
is responsible that the labels referred to in Appendix II are
attached to animals before they are handed over.

2. He will immediately bring to the notice of commanders of
units any points which may bear upon the health and condition,
or affect wastage of the animals under his professional care.

3. He must be ever on the alert to prevent the introduction or
spread of contagious diseases ; he will make frequent and careful
inspections, which should be carried out as opportunities are
afforded by the military situation.

4. He will inspect all horses joining the unit, and will immediately
report all suspicious cases and outbreaks of contagious disease
to commanders of units and to the Assistant Director of Veterinary
Services of the formation.

5. Every Friday he will send the Assistant Director of Veterinary
Services a weekly return (Army Form A 2000) of sick and injured
animals in the units under his care. This return will include
casualties up to Thursday evening. He will keep a record in
Army Book 32 of all cases treated.

6. All requisitions for veterinary stores will be submitted through
the Assistant Director of Veterinary Services.

6. OFFICERS ATTACHED TO REMOUNT DEPOTS.

Officers, Army Veterinary Corps, are attached to Remount
Depots as shown in War Establishments ; their duties are analogous
to those laid down in Section 5 for officers attached to units.
They correspond directly with the Director of Veterinary Services or
his representative on the Lines of Communication on all technical
matters.

7. OFFICERS ALLOTTED TO THE ADJUTANT-GENERAL'S OFFICE AT THE BASE.

1. An Officer, Army Veterinary Corps, will be allotted to the
Adjutant-General's office at the Base to deal with correspondence

and documents relating to the Army Veterinary Corps personnel engaged in the campaign. He will receive his instructions through the Deputy Adjutant-General at the base.

2. He will prepare the veterinary statistics from information supplied by the Assistant Director of Veterinary Services of formations and Officers Commanding Veterinary Hospitals.

3. He will submit such periodical consolidated returns as may be desired by the Secretary of the War Office.

8. VETERINARY ESTABLISHMENTS WITH UNITS.

1. Veterinary officers are allotted to units as laid down in War Establishments.

2. Veterinary arrangements for units for whom no veterinary officer is provided will be made by the Assistant Director of Veterinary Services of the division, but when these units are in brigade areas they will be in charge of the veterinary officer attached to the headquarters of the infantry brigade quartered in the brigade area. On the line of march or in emergency they will apply to the nearest veterinary officer.

9. MOBILE VETERINARY SECTIONS.

1. Mobile veterinary sections are field units, one being allotted to each division and Cavalry Brigade. Their personnel is laid down in War Establishments.

2. Their function is to take charge of sick and injured animals sent to them under proper authority and convey them to veterinary hospitals.

3. Subject to the orders of divisional commanders, their movements are controlled by the Assistant Director of Veterinary Services of the formation.

4. Sick and injured animals are despatched from railhead in the returning supply train. The officer commanding mobile veterinary section will report to the railhead commandant, who will detail trucks for the purpose.

5. A conducting party of one man per truck and one N.C.O. in charge will be sent with each consignment, every man being provided with a canvas bucket for watering on route.

6. A statement in duplicate (as pro-forma Appendix III) showing number of horses transferred, will be sent with the conducting party, one copy being signed by the receiving officer and returned as a receipt.

7. All cases will be dressed and attended to previous to despatch. Particular attention is to be given to the provision of sufficient fodder for the journey, and that animals are securely tied up.

8. The officer commanding the receiving hospital is responsible for the return of the conducting party without delay. On reaching railhead the party will travel on the supply column lorries to refilling point, from thence rejoining sections.

9. On despatch of each consignment, the officer commanding mobile veterinary section will notify by wire the Deputy-Director of Veterinary Services of Army or Cavalry Corps concerned, and officer commanding receiving hospital, giving numbers and date.

10. In the case of Mange, truck numbers will be included in these wires, and rugs and blankets of the horses will accompany them to the hospital.

11. When the division is stationary, the mobile veterinary section will also act as a temporary hospital for selected cases which may recover before further movement is ordered. Considerable discretion must be shown in choosing suitable cases for retention under the circumstances, and when cured they will be returned to units.

12. The N.C.O. in charge of a returning conducting party will be responsible for the drawing and conveyance of any veterinary stores required by the formation to which his mobile veterinary section is attached.

10. VETERINARY HOSPITALS.

1. Veterinary hospitals, allotted on a scale proportionate to the strength of the Armies in the Field, are stationary units located on the Lines of Communication, at such places as circumstances indicate advisable.

2. The personnel is as laid down in War Establishments.

3. All sick and injured animals will be transferred to them for treatment, and when cured will be handed over to the nearest remount depot.

4. The situation of a veterinary hospital will depend on the local conditions, and advantage should be taken of existing buildings whenever available which could be adapted to the requirements of a veterinary hospital in providing shelter from the weather for sick and debilitated animals. When no buildings can be utilized, the hospital will be laid out on a plan suggested by the Director of Veterinary Services in co-operation with the Director of Works, and approved by the I.G.C.

5. The choice of site should also be dependent on its accessibility to the railway station or siding at which sick animals consigned to it would be detrained, an adequate water supply, and facilities for obtaining supplies and forage.

6. In all hospitals suitable provision should be made to ensure efficient isolation of animals suspicious of or suffering from

contagious disease. Outbreaks of the latter will be at once reported to the Director of Veterinary Services, the source of infection being stated.

7. The officer commanding is responsible for the sanitary condition of the hospital and quarters or localities occupied by the personnel, and will arrange for a systematic disposal of refuse and carcases of animals dying in hospital by burning or other methods. He will make arrangements for detachments to meet sick animals arriving by rail.

8. He will furnish the returns laid down in Field Service Regulations, Part II, for commanders of units, He will also furnish to the Director of Veterinary Services daily (by noon) a telegram giving the alterations in strength under the following headings:—

"Admitted," "Died," "Destroyed," "Cast and Sold," "Cured," and "Remaining under Treatment,"

a duplicate of which should be sent to Officer i/c Army Veterinary Records at the base, and a weekly return, on Army Form A 2000, made up to Thursday evening.

11. VETERINARY CONVALESCENT DEPOTS.

1. One or more veterinary convalescent depots will be located on the Lines of Communication, as circumstances indicate. They are intended for the reception of such cases as require only rest and good feeding.

2. Arrangements for these, whether in open fields or kraals, will depend upon climatic conditions, or upon the feasibility of obtaining land suitable for the purpose.

3. The personnel will be as laid down in War Establishments.

12. DEPOTS FOR VETERINARY STORES.

1. A base depot of veterinary stores as laid down in War Establishment will be located at the base, and an advanced depot will be attached to the advanced or receiving veterinary hospital. Both of these depots will be administered by the Director of Veterinary Services.

2. The officer in charge of the base depot of veterinary stores will submit to the Director of Veterinary Services requisitions necessary to keep the stocks up to requirements.

3. The officer in charge of the base depot will comply with indents received from the officer in charge of advanced depot, and also from the officer commanding veterinary hospitals on the Lines of Communication. Any abnormal demand will be referred to the Director of Veterinary Services for such action as may be necessary.

4. The officer in charge of the advanced depot of veterinary stores will deal with the indents received from Assistant Directors of Veterinary Services of formations, the stores being conveyed to the formations by means of returning horse-conducting parties of mobile veterinary sections.

5. No local purchase of veterinary stores will be made except by special authority of the Director of Veterinary Services. Purchase or sale by units is prohibited.

13. SUPPLY OF VETERINARY STORES.

1. Arrangements will be made for the despatch to the theatre of war of a supply of veterinary stores and equipment which is calculated to last three months.

2. The Director of Veterinary Services is responsible for the maintenance of sufficient stocks in the theatre of operations to meet requirements. He should utilize any available local sources of supply. Demands for stores from home should be made sufficiently in advance to admit of them arriving at the base as required.

14. AUDIT OF ACCOUNTS.

1. Accounts will only be rendered for base depots and advanced depots from which stores are issued in bulk. The accounts will be kept in Army Book 169, a detail being kept of all stores received. Receipts will be taken on charge immediately the articles are delivered, and the vouchers filed. All issues from these depots to veterinary hospitals, &c., will be treated as final. Entries in the accounts will be supported by receipted vouchers where possible. If, owing to exceptional circumstances due to war conditions (which should be explained), receipted vouchers cannot be obtained, evidence that the articles were indented for and despatched should be obtained and put up with the account in support of the issue.

2. The accounts will be balanced half-yearly, or as mutually arranged between the Director of Veterinary Services and the local auditor, and will be forwarded to the latter for audit not later than the end of the month following the date of closing.

3. Stock is to be taken from time to time as circumstances permit by the officer in charge of a depot. Immediately after the termination of hostilities, boards of officers will be appointed to take stock of stores of every description at the depots. The officer in charge of a depot will previously balance his account up to the date of stocktaking, and the board will count personally the articles in possession. The articles thus counted will be entered as " Stock on (date) " by the officer in charge, in a line below the " Remain " in his account, and the correctness of the quantities

as shown will be certified by the Stocktaking Board. The discrepancies between the " Remain " and " Stock " will be shown by the officer in charge, the surpluses in one line and the deficiencies in another below the " Stock." The account will then be rendered for audit, accompanied by the proceedings of the board, and a statement from the officer in charge giving an explanation of the discrepancies, together with the recommendation of the Director of Veterinary Services.

4. A new or " peace " depot will also be started, such stores as are in good condition and required for issue being separated from the old or " war " depot stock and transferred by voucher to a " peace " account. The officer in charge of the old depot will be held responsible, as far as the exigencies of the service permit, for the old depot account until the stock is disposed of. Any stores which may be considered as unfit for issue will be dealt with in accordance with Regulations.

5. In the case of veterinary stores in hospitals and with units, &c., similar stocktakings will be made, and the stores remaining immediately brought on charge in the ordinary " peace " accounts. All veterinary stores not required for current use will then be returned to the nearest depot, and struck off in the account supported by the usual vouchers.

APPENDIX I.

FIELD SERVICE.

A.F. A 2000.

Corps, &c.

Return of Sick and Injured Animals During the Week Ending

Station _____ Date _____

	In last Return.	Admitted since.	Total.	*Cured.	Transferred Sick.	Transferred C.H. Depôt.	Died.	Destroyed.	Cast and Sold.	Remaining under Treatment.	Total.	Remarks (nature of cases to be stated).
1. General diseases ...												
2. Respiratory diseases ...												
3. Circulatory ,, ...												
4. Urinary ,, ...												
5. Generative ,, ...												
6. Digestive ,, ...												
7. Lymphatic ,, ...												
8. Nervous ,, ...												
9. Skin ,, ...												
10. Locomotory ,, ...												
11. Specific ,, ...												
12. Visual ,, ...												
13. Injuries												

* Number transferred cured to remount depôts to be also noted in column of Remarks.

Present Strength of Animals. { Horses ....
Mules ....

Total _____

Veterinary Officer.

Personnel of Hospital.
(To be completed by Os.C. Hospitals only.)

(A.V.C. and Cavalry Staff Reservists.)	Effective.	Non-Effective.	Attached.	Effective.	Non-Effective.
Warrant Officer ...					
Staff-Serjts. & Serjts.					
Corporals					
Privates					
Farrier Q.M.S., Staff-Serjts. & Serjts. ...					
Corporal S.-Smiths ...					
Shoeing-Smiths ...					
Saddler Corporals ...					
Saddler...					
Total ...					

Veterinary Officers of Formations or Hospitals.

Rank.	Name.	Charge.	Rank.	Name.	Charge.

Contagious Disease.
Remarks as to action taken.

APPENDIX II.

Labels for attachment to sick and injured animals sent from units of the Field Army to Veterinary Hospitals L. of C. and referred to in paragraph 1, Section 5 :—

White	...	Medical cases.
Green	...	Surgical ,,
Red	...	Specific ,,
Blue	...	For cast horses other than veterinary cases.

```
       ARMY VETERINARY SERVICE.

   Unit ...........................................
O  Disease ......................................
            .........................v. o.
```

APPENDIX III.

Pro-Forma.

Herewith.......................horses (sick) of........... ....unit

of formation, in charge of........... ....and ....men.

The N.C.O. and men have been rationed up to and for........................

The horses have been rationed up to and for.... .. ..

Kindly acknowledge receipt of horses hereon, and return by N.C.O. i/c Conducting Party.

Signature.

Place.

Date.

LONDON:
PRINTED FOR HIS MAJESTY'S STATIONERY OFFICE,
By HARRISON AND SONS, ST. MARTIN'S LANE,
PRINTERS IN ORDINARY TO HIS MAJESTY.

(As to prices in brackets, see top of page 2.)

GUNS. Drill for—*continued.*

6-inch B.L. Marks VII. and VII^v. Land Service. 1914. 1*d.* (1*d.*)
6-inch B.L. Howitzer. 1912. (Reprinted, with Amendments to Dec. 1914). 1*d.* (1*d.*)
6-inch Q.F. Land Service. 1914. 1*d.* (1*d.*)
5-inch B.L. Howitzer. 1912. (Reprinted, 1914, with Amendments). 1*d.* (1*d.*)
4·7-inch Q.F. Fixed Armament. Land Service. 1914. 1*d.* (1*d.*)
4·7-inch Q.F., on Travelling Carriages. 1912. 1*d.* (1*d.*)
4·7-inch Q.F. Heavy Batteries. Provisional. 1914. 1*d.* (1*d.*)
4·5-inch Q.F. Howitzer. 1914. 1*d.* (1*d.*)
4-inch Q.F. Land Service. 1914. 1*d.* (1*d.*)
2·95-inch Q.F. 1914. 1*d.* (1*d.*)

GUNS. Handbooks for. (*And see* **GUNS.** Drill for):—

60-pr. B.L. Land Service. 1913. 1*s.* 6*d.* (1*s.* 3*d.*)
18-pr. Q.F. Land Service. 1913. (Reprinted, with Amendments, 1914). 1*s.* (11*d.*)
15-pr. B.L. Marks II. to IV., and Carriages, Marks II.* and IV., and Wagon. and Limber. Mark IV. Field Batteries. 1914. Provisional. 1*s.* (10*d.*)
15-pr. B.L.C. Marks I., II., II.*, and IV., with Mark I. Carriage, and Marks I., I*a.*, I*b.*, and I*c.* Limbers and Wagons. Land Service. 1912. 1*s.* (10*d.*)
15-pr. Q.F. Land Service. 1914. 1*s.* 6*d.* (1*s.* 2*d.*)
13-pr. Q.F. Land Service. 1913. (Reprinted, with Amendments, 1914.) 1*s.* 3*d.* (1*s.* 1*d.*)
12-pr. B.L. of 6 cwt. Marks I. to IV. and IV*a.* and Carriages Marks I.* I.**, and II. Horse Artillery. 1905. 1*s.* (11*d.*)
10-pr. Jointed B.L. Mule Equipment. 1914. 1*s.* 6*d.* (1*s.* 2*d.*)
9·45-inch B.L. Howitzer. 1906. 9*d.* (7*d.*)
9·2-inch B.L. Mark IX., "C" Mark IX., and Marks X., X^v., and X.* Land Service. 1912. 1*s.* (11*d.*)
8-inch R.M.L. Howitzer of 70 cwt. Movable Armament and Armament of Works. Land Service. 1901. 2*s.* (1*s.* 6*d.*)
6-inch B.L. and B.L.C. Guns, Mountings, &c. 1904. 1*s.* 6*d.* (1*s.* 4*d.*)
6-inch B.L. Marks VII. and VII^v. Land Service. 1911. 9*d.* (8*d.*)
(*Under revision*)
6-inch B.L. 30 cwt. Howitzer. Marks I. and I.* 1915. 1*s.* 6*d.* (*In the press*)
6-inch Q.F. Land Service. 1903. 1*s.* (10*d.*)
6-inch "B" Q.F. Land Service. 1911. 1*s.* (10*d.*)
5·4-inch B.L. Howitzer. Mark. I. 1902. 1*s.* 6*d.* (1*s.* 2*d.*)
5-inch B.L. Marks I.—V. 1904. 9*d.* (9*d.*)
5-inch B.L. Marks IV.—V. Land Service. 1903. 1*s.* 6*d.* (1*s.* 2*d.*)
5-inch B.L. Howitzer. 1915. (*In the press*)
4·7-inch Q.F. Fixed Armaments. Land Service. 1904. 1*s.* (11*d.*)
4·7-inch Q.F.B., on Travelling Carriages. Land Service. 1910. (Reprinted, with Amendments, 1914). 9*d.* (8*d.*)
4·5-inch Q.F. Howitzer. Land Service. 1914. 1*s.* 3*d.* (1*s.* 1*d.*)
2·95-inch Q.F. Mule Equipment and Man Transport Equipment. 1914. 2*s.* (1*s.* 6*d.*)
·803-inch Vickers Machine (Magazine Rifle Chamber), on Tripod Mounting, Mark IV. 1914. 6*d.* (6*d.*)
0·803-inch Nordenfelt 3-barrel and Gardner 2-barrel converted from 0·4-inch and 0·45-inch M.H. Chamber, Magazine Rifle Chamber, on Carriages, 1900. 9*d.* (8*d.*)

HISTORICAL RECORDS OF THE BRITISH ARMY, viz.:—

Horse Guards. 5*s.* (3*s.* 7*d.*)
Dragoon Guards, 3rd, 4th, 5th, 6th, and 7th. Each 4*s.* (3*s.*)

(As to prices in brackets, see top of p ge 2.)

Historical Records—*continued*.
>Dragoons, 1st, 3rd, 7th, 14th, and 16th.   Each 4s.   (3s.)
>>Ditto.   12th, and 13th.   Each 3s.   (2s. 3d.)
>Marine Corps.   3s.   (2s. 2d.)
>Foot, 2nd, 6th, 8th, 10th, 11th, 13th. 16th, 17th, 18th. 19th, 20th, 21st, 22nd, 34th, 36th, 39th. 46th, 53rd, 67th, 71st, 72nd, 73rd, 74th, 86th, 87th, and 92nd.   Each 4s.   (3s.)
>· Do. 14th, 56th, 61st, 70th, and 88th.   Each 3s.   (2s. 3d.)

HISTORIES, SHORT, OF THE TERRITORIAL REGIMENTS OF THE BRITISH ARMY.   67 numbers, each 1d.   In one volume, 5s.   (3s. 9d.)
>Ditto.   The Scots Guards.   1d.   (1d.)
>Ditto.   The 6th (Inniskilling) Dragoons.   1d.   (1d.)
>Ditto.   Revised Editions.   1d.   (1d.) each :—

Alexandra, Princess of Wales's Own (Yorkshire Regiment).
The Bedfordshire Regiment.
The Black Watch (Royal Highlanders).
The Cameronians (Scottish Rifles).
The Cheshire Regiment.
The Duke of Wellington's West Riding Regiment.
The Durham Light Infantry.
The East Lancashire Regiment.
The East Surrey Regiment.
The Hampshire Regiment.
The Highland Light Infantry.
The King's Own Yorkshire Light Infantry.
The Lancashire Fusiliers.
The Loyal North Lancashire Regiment.
The Northamptonshire Regiment.
The Oxfordshire and Buckinghamshire Light Infantry.
The Prince Albert's (Somersetshire Light Infantry).
The Prince of Wales's Leinster Regiment (Royal Canadians).
The Prince of Wales's Volunteers (South Lancashire Regiment).
The Princess Charlotte of Wales's (The Royal Berkshire Regiment).
The Princess Louise's Argyll and Sutherland Highlanders.
The Royal Inniskilling Fusiliers.
The Royal Sussex Regiment.
The Royal Warwickshire Regiment.
The Royal Welsh Fusiliers.
The Suffolk Regiment.
The Welsh Regiment.

HOSPITALS. MILITARY FAMILIES'.   Nursing Staff Regulations, Dec., 1909.   1d.   (1d.)

HOSTILITIES WITHOUT DECLARATION OF WAR FROM 1700 TO 1870.   2s.   (1s. 7d.)

HYGIENE. ELEMENTARY MILITARY.   Manual of.   1912.   6d.   (6d.)

INDIAN EMPIRE. OUR.   A Short Review and some Hints for the use of Soldiers proceeding to India.   6d.   (6d.)

INFANTRY TRAINING.   (4-Company Organization.)   1914.   6d.   (6d.)

INSTITUTES. Garrison and Regimental.   Rules for the Management of.   1912.   1d.   (1d.)

INTELLIGENCE DUTIES IN THE FIELD.   Regns. for.   1904.   2d.   (2d.)

ITALIAN CAVALRY TRAINING REGULATIONS. 1911.   Training for Marches, Tactics of Minor Units, and Training of Patrols.   Translated.   4d.   (3d.)

JAMAICA.   Standing Orders.   1912.   1s.   (9d.)

JERSEY. ROYAL MILITIA OF THE ISLAND OF.   Regulations.   1914.   With the Jersey Militia Law, 1905.   1s. 3d.   (11d.)

KING'S REGULATIONS AND ORDERS FOR THE ARMY. , 1912.   (Reprinted, with Amendments published in Army Orders up to Aug. 1, 1914).   1s   (1s.)

(As to prices in brackets, see top of page 2.)

KIT PLATES :—
    Artillery. Royal—
        1. Horse and Field. Kit in Barrack Room. 1912. 2*d.* (2*d.*)
        2.   Ditto.   Kit laid out for Inspection. 1903. 2*d.* (2*d.*)
        6. Garrison. Kit laid out for Inspection. 1909. 2*d.* (2*d.*)
      10. Ditto. Kit in Barrack Room. 1909. 2*d.* (2*d.*)
    Cavalry. 1891. 1*d.* (1*d.*)
    Engineers. Royal—
        1. Dismounted. Detail of Shelf and Bedding, with Marching Order ready
          to put on. Detail of Shelf and Bedding, with Drill Order ready to
          put on. 1914. 1*d.* (1*d.*)
        2. Dismounted. Full Kit laid out for Inspection in Barrack Room.
          1914. 1*d.* (1*d.*)
        4. Mounted N.C.O. or Driver and Field Troop Sapper. Full Kit laid out
          for Inspection in Barrack Room. 1910. 1*d.* (1*d.*)
        5. Mounted. Detail of Shelf and Bedding. 1910. 1*d.* (1*d.*)
        6. Driver, with pair of Horses. Field Kit laid out for Inspection or Parade,
          including Articles carried in Valise on Baggage Wagon. 1899. 1*d.*
          (1*d.*)
    Infantry—
        1. Kit in Barrack Room. 1905. 2*d.* (2*d.*)
        2. Kit laid out for inspection. 1905. 2*d.* (2*d.*)
      Highland. 1884. 1*d.* (1*d.*)
    Medical Corps. Royal Army. Kit in Barrack Room. 1912. 2*d.* (2*d.*)
    Ordnance Corps. Army. For guidance at Marching Order and Kit
      Inspections. 2*d.* (2*d.*)

LARGE FORMATIONS. The Operations of. (Conduite des Grandes
    Unités). Translated from the Field Service Regulations of the French
    Army, dated Oct. 28, 1913. 6*d.* (5*d.*)

LAW. Military. Manual of. 1914. 2*s.* (1*s.* 9*d.*)

LAW FOR THE RESERVE FORCES AND MILITIA. Manual of.
    1886. 1*s.* 6*d.* (1*s.* 2*d.*)

MACHINE-GUN. Tests of Elementary Training. 1*d.* (1*d.*)

MACHINE GUNS AND SMALL ARMS, ·303-inch. Nomenclature of
    Parts. Stripping. Assembling, Action, Jams, Missfires. Failures. and
    Inspection of. Revised Edition. 1913. 3*d.* (3*d.*); Amendments, No. 1.
    1*d.* (1*d.*)

MAGAZINES AND CARE OF WAR MATÉRIEL. Regulations for.
    1913. 9*d.* (9*d.*); Amendments, July 1914. 1*d.* (1*d.*)

MAP READING AND FIELD SKETCHING. Manual. 1912. (Re-
    printed, with Additions, 1914). 1*s.* (11*d.*) (*And see* Schools, Army.)

MECHANISM AS APPLIED TO ARTILLERY. Notes on. Second
    edition. 1902. 1*s.* (11*d.*)

MEDICAL CORPS. Royal Army (*and see* Territorial Force):—
    Admission to. Regulations for. Jan. 1912. 1*d.* (1*d.*)
    Standing Orders. 1914. 1*s.* (10*d.*)
    Training. 1911. 9*d.* (9*d.*)

MEDICAL DEPARTMENT. Army. Index to Appendices of Reports
    from 1859 to 1896. 3*d.* (3*d.*)

MEDICAL SERVICE. Army. Regulations. 1906. (Reprinted, with
    Amendments up to Sept. 1914). 4*d.* (5*d.*)

MEDICAL SERVICE. Strategical and Tactical Employment of the, as
    carried out in an Army Corps; with a series of Problems. Translated
    from the Austrian. 4*s.* 6*d.* (3*s.* 4*d.*)

(As to prices in brackets, see top of page 2.)

MEDICAL SERVICES. Army. Advisory Board for. The Treatment of Venereal Disease **and** Scabies. First Report. 1904. 1*s.* 6*d.* (1*s.* 3*d.*); Second Report. 1905. 2*s.* (1*s.* 6*d.*); Third Report. 1905. 1*s.* (10*d.*); Final Report. 1906. 6*d.* (5*d.*)

MEDICAL SERVICES OF FOREIGN ARMIES. Handbook of. Part I. FRANCE. 6*d.* (5*d.*) (*Under revision*); Part II. GERMANY. 6*d.* (5*d.*); Part III. AUSTRIA-HUNGARY. 6*d.* (5*d.*); Part IV. RUSSIA. 6*d.* (5*d.*); Part V. ITALY. 6*d.* (5*d.*); Part VI. THE NETHERLANDS AND BELGIUM. 1911. 6*d.* (5*d.*)

MEKOMETER. Handbook. 1911. 6*d.* (6*d.*)

MUSKETRY REGULATIONS:—
Part I. 1909. (Reprinted, with Amendments, 1914). 6*d.* (7*d.*)
Part II. Rifle Ranges and Musketry Appliances. 1910. (Reprinted, with Amendments to Oct. 31, 1914). 4*d.* (4*d.*)

NIGHT OPERATIONS. Elementary Training in. 1911. 1*d.* (1*d.*)

NUMBER OF TROOPS TO THE YARD in the Principal Battles since 1850. Memo. on. With opinions of Modern Authorities on limits of extension at the present day. 1884. 9*d.* (7*d.*)

NURSING IN THE ARMY. Queen Alexandra's Imperial Military Nursing Service. Reprinted from " The British Medical Journal." 1905. 1*d.* (1*d.*)

NURSING SERVICE. Queen Alexandra's Imperial Military. Regulations for Admission to the. 1914. 1*d.* (1*d.*)

OFFICERS TRAINING CORPS:—
Regulations. 1912. 2*d.* (2*d.*)   (*Under revision*)
Ditto.   (Inns of Court). 1*d.* (1*d.*)
Special A.O., March 16, 1908. 1*d.* (1*d.*)
Junior Division. Instruction for the Annual Camps. 1913. 2*d.* (2*d.*)

OPERATION ORDERS. A Technical Study by Hans von Kiesling. Translated from the German. 1*s.* 6*d.* (1*s.* 3*d.*)

OPTICAL MANUAL or Handbook of Instructions for the guidance of Surgeons. Third edition. 1885. 1*s.* 6*d.* (1*s.* 3*d.*)

OPTICS. Notes on. 6*d.* (5*d.*)

ORANGE FREE STATE. Topographical Survey of the, 1905-1911. Report on the. 10*s.* (7*s.*)

ORDNANCE COLLEGE (*and see* Artillery College):—
Advanced Classes. Reports on (up to the 33rd). Each 1*s.* (9*d.*)
Ditto. 34th. 6*d.* (5*d.*)
Dynamics. Notes on. Second edition. 3*s.* (2*s.* 5*s.*)
Officers' Mess (Royal Artillery) Management and First Principles of Book-keeping. 3*d.* (3*d.*)
Ordnance Courses. Reports on. Each 1*s.* (9*d.*)
Regulations. 1907. 2*d.* (2*d.*)

ORDNANCE CORPS. Army. Standing Orders. 1912. (Reprinted, with Amendments to June 30, 1914). 6*d.* (6*d.*)   (*In the press*)

ORDNANCE MANUAL (WAR). 1914. 6*d.* (5*d.*)

ORDNANCE. SERVICE. Treatise on. Seventh edition. 1908. With volume of plates. 7*s.* 6*d.* (5*s.* 6*d.*); Amendments. June 1909. Dec. 1910, Dec. 1912. Each 1*d.* (1*d.*); Ditto. Dec. 1909, Dec. 1911. Each 2*d.* (2*d.*)

ORDNANCE SERVICES. ARMY. Regulations :—
Part I. 1912. (Reprinted, with Amendments published in Army Orders up to Oct. 1, 1914). 6*d.* (6*d.*)
Part II. 1914. Instructions for Laboratories and Laboratory Operations, Examination of Explosives and Ordnance. 1*s.* (11*d.*)

PATHOLOGICAL SPECIMENS in the Museum of the Army Medical Department, Netley. Descriptive Catalogue of. Third edition. Vol. 1. By Sir W. Aitken, M.D. 1892. 5*s.* (3*s.* 8*d.*)

14

(As to prices in brackets, see top of page 2.)

PAY DUTIES of Officers Commanding Squadrons, Batteries, Companies, &c. Instructions. 1914. 1*d.* (1*d.*) *(Under revision)*

PHYSICAL TRAINING. Manual of. (Reprint 1908 with Amendments published in Army Orders to Dec. 1, 1914). 9*d.* (9*d.*)

PLACE-NAMES OCCURRING ON FOREIGN MAPS. Rules for the Transliteration of. 1906. 1*s.* (9*d.*)

PORTABLE SUB-TARGET (Mark I.), and How to Use it. 1911. (Reprinted, with Amendments, 1914.) 1*d.* (1*d.*)

POSTAL SERVICES. ARMY. WAR. Manual of. 1913. 3*d.* (3*d.*)

PROJECTION, &c. Linear Perspective. A Text-Book for use of the R.M. Academy. Part I.—Text. Part II.—Plates. 1904. 6*s.* (4*s.* 5*d.*)

PUBLICATIONS (RECENT) OF MILITARY INTEREST. List of, Quarterly. Nos. 1 to 8. 2*d.* (2*d.*) each; Nos. 9 to 17. 4*d.* (4*d.*) each. *(Continued by* THE ARMY REVIEW).

RAILWAY DISTANCES. Ireland. Handbook of. Third edition. 1884. 7*s.* 6*d.* (5*s.* 3*d.*)

RAILWAY MANUAL (WAR). 1911. (Reprinted, with Amendments, 1914). 6*d.* (5*d.*)

RAILWAYS. MILITARY. RECONNAISSANCE AND SURVEY OF. Notes on, for Officers of R.E. Railway Companies. 1910. 2*s.* 3*d.* (1*s.* 8*d.*)

RANGE-FINDER. Handbooks:—
Infantry, No. 1. (Marindin). 1913. 3*d.* (3*d.*)
Infantry, No. 2. (Barr and Stroud). 31·5-inches base. 1913. 1*s.* (10*d.*)
Watkin. Regulations for instruction in, and practice with. 1882. 1*s.* (9*d.*)

RANGE FINDING. COAST DEFENCE. Manual of. Part I. 9*d.* (8*d.*)
Ditto. Amendments, June 30, 1914. 1*d.* (1*d.*)

RANGES, MINIATURE CARTRIDGE. *(Reprinted from* THE ARMY REVIEW, January 1914). 3*d.* (3*d.*)

RECRUITING FOR THE REGULAR ARMY AND THE SPECIAL RESERVE. Regulations. 1912. (Reprinted, with Amendments to Aug. 31, 1914). 3*d.* (3*d.*)

REMOUNT MANUAL (WAR). 1913. 2*d.* (2*d.*)

REMOUNT REGULATIONS. 1913. 3*d.* (3*d.*)

REQUISITIONING OF SUPPLIES, TRANSPORT, STORES, ANIMALS, LABOUR, &c., IN THE FIELD. Instructions for the. 1907. 1*d.* (1*d.*)

RESERVE *(and see* Motor Reserve; Special Reserve):—
Army Reserve. Class I. Regulations. 1911. 1*d.* (1*d.*)
Ditto. Amendments, June 1913. 1*d.* (1*d.*)
National Reserve. Regulations. 1913. 1*d.* (1*d.*)

RIFLE RANGES. Care and Construction of. Instructions for. 1908. 3*d.* (3*d.*)

RIFLE RANGES, TRAINING GROUND, AND MUSKETRY CAMP, PENALLY. (Western Coast Defences.) Standing Orders. 1910. 2*d.* (2*d.*)

RIFLES, &c. Cleaning of. Notes on the. 1911. 25 for 6*d.* (7*d.*)

RIFLES, SHORT AND CHARGER-LOADING, MAGAZINE, LEE-ENFIELD. Handbook for Serjeant-Instructors of Special Reserve, Officers Training Corps, and Territorial Force in regard to the Care, Inspection, &c., of. 3*d.* (3*d.*)

RUSSIAN MILITARY AND NAVAL TERMS. Dictionary of. 1906. 3*s.* 6*d.* (2*s.* 6*d.*)

RUSSO-JAPANESE WAR :—
Medical and Sanitary Reports from Officers attached to the Japanese and Russian Forces in the Field. 1908. 5*s.* (3*s.* 10*d.*)

(As to prices in brackets, see top of page 2.)

Russo-Japanese War—*continued.*

Official History. Part I. Causes of the War. Opening Events up to and including the Battle of the Ya-lu. Second edition. 1909. **1s. 6d.** (1s. 3d.); Part II From the Battle of the Ya-lu to Liao-yang, exclusive. 1908. 5s. (3s. 8d.); Part III. The Siege of Port Arthur. 1909. 4s. 6d. (3s. 4d.); Part IV. Liao-yang. 1910. 4s. (3s.); Part V. Sha Ho. 1911. 4s. 6d. (3s. 5d.)

Official History (Naval and Military). Vol. I. To August 24, 1904. With case of Maps. 1910. 15s. (10s. 7d.); Vol. II. Liao-yang, the Sha-ho, Port Arthur. With case of Maps. 1912. 15s. (10s. 10d.)

Reports from British Officers attached to the Japanese and Russian Forces in the Field. In three vols., with two cases of Maps (*not sold separately*). 21s. (15s.)

SALISBURY PLAIN. SOUTHERN COMMAND. Standing Orders applicable to all Troops Encamped on Salisbury Plain, and applicable generally to Troops Quartered at Bulford and Tidworth. 1913. 3d. (3d.)

"SAM-BROWNE" BELT, SCABBARD, AND SWORD KNOT. Specification and Drawings. 1899. 1d. (1d.)

SCHOOLS. Army:—

Annual Reports on. 1911-12; 1912-13. Each 1s. (9d.)

Map Reading. Notes on. 1915. 3d. (3d.)
(*And see* Map Reading and Field Sketching.)

Military and other Terms, and Words which Occur in Orders. Lists of. 1914. 2d. (2d.)

Physiology. Elementary. Handbook. 1901. 1d. (1d.)

Regulations. 1911. 4d. (4d.)

School Hygiene. Handbook of. For Teachers. 6d. (6d.)

Singing in. Regns. for Teaching. 1911. 1d. (1d.)

Standing Orders for Inspectors, Examiners, and Teachers. 1910. 6d. (5d.)

Type Exercises of Extracts from Regimental Orders for the use of Candidates for Third-class Certificates of Education. 1912. 3d. (3d.)

SCOUTS. Training and Use of. Lecture by Col. F. C. Carter. 1905. 2d. (2d.)

SCREWS. Standard Leading. Provision of, for Screw-cutting Lathes. Report of Committee. 1905. 1s. (10d.)

SEVASTOPOL. Siege of. 1854-55. 3 vols., with Case of Maps and Plans. Half Mor., £5 4s. Cloth, £4 4s.
Or separately:—Vol. I. Engineer Operations. £1 6s.; Vol. II. Ditto. With Case of Maps and Plans. £2 10s.; Vol. III. Artillery Operations. 10s.

SEWAGE. Practical Treatment of. The latest development of. 1903. 6d. (5d.)

SHOEBURYNESS GARRISON. Standing Orders. 1913. 1s. 6d. (1s. 1d.)

SIEGE OPERATIONS in the Campaign against France, 1870-71. (*Von Tiedemann.*) Translated. 4s. 6d. (3s. 3d.)

SIGNALLING. Training Manual. 1907. (Reprinted, with Amendments to May 1, 1911). (*Out of print*); Amendments. Nov. 1912, May 1913, April and Aug. 1914 (in one). Each 1d. (1d.); Appendix IV. Despatch Riding. 1d. (1d.)

SIGNALLING. Training Manual. Part II. For the use of the Divisional Signal Companies and Intercommunication Personnel of Units in Divisions, other than 1st to 8th Divisions, of the Intercommunication Personnel of Units of the Territorial Force other than Signal Units and R.G.A. Coast Defence Companies, and of Signallers of King Edward's Horse. 1914. 6d. (5d.)

Ditto. Appendix I. Telephone Cable Drill. Artillery. 1d. (1d.)

Ditto. Appendix II. Telegraph Cable Drill. 2d. (2d.)

Ditto. Appendix III. Telephone Equipment. Artillery Batteries and Infantry Battalions. 1d. (1d.)

Ditto. Amendments. April 1915. 1d. (1d.)

16

(As to prices in brackets, see top of page 2.)

SIGNALLING DISC. Directions for Use. 1911. 1*d.* (1*d.*)

SIGNAL SERVICE. THE ARMY. 1*d.* (1*d.*)

SIGNAL SERVICE. ARMY. Manual of—WAR. Provisional. 1914. 2*d.* (2*d.*)

SMALL ARMS Text Book. 1909. With Tables. 2*s.* 6*d.* (2*s.* 1*d.*)

SMALL WARS. Their Principles and Practice. Third Edition. 1906. (*Reprinted* 1909.) 4*s.* (3*s.*)

SOMALILAND :—

    Military Report on. 1907. Vol. I. Geographical, Descriptive, and Historical. 2*s.* (1*s.* 7*d.*)

    Operations in, 1901-04. Official History. Vol. I. 3*s.* (2*s.* 4*d.*); Vol. II. 4*s.* (3*s.*)

SOUTH AFRICAN WAR, 1899-1902 :—

    Medical Arrangements. 7*s.* 6*d.* (5*s.* 6*d.*)

    Medical History. An Epidemiological Essay. [Reprinted from " The Journal of the Royal Army Medical Corps."] 3*s.* 9*d.* (2*s.* 9*d.*)

    Railways. 4*s.* (3*s.*)

    Surgical Cases Noted. 7*s.* 6*d.* (5*s.* 6*d.*)

    Telegraph Operations. 10*s.* (7*s.* 1*d.*)

    Voluntary Organizations in aid of the Sick and Wounded. Report of the Central British Red Cross Committee on. 1902. 3*s.* (2*s.* 5*d.*)

SPECIAL RESERVE :—

    Commission in the Special Reserve of Officers. Short Guide to obtaining a ; &c. 1*d.* (1*d.*)

    Regulations for Officers of the Special Reserve of Officers, and for the Special Reserve. 1911. 4*d.* (5*d.*)

    Scheme for the Provision, Organization, and Training of the Special Reserve required to supplement the Regular Army, and the Application of the Scheme to the existing Militia. (Special A.O., Dec. 23, 1907.) 2*d.* (2*d.*)

    Scheme for the Provision, Organization, and Training of that portion which will be drawn from the Territorial Force to supplement the Regular Army on Mobilization being ordered. (Special A.O., Nov. 20, 1908.) 2*d.* (2*d.*)

STAFF COLLEGE Regulations (Camberley). 1905. Reprinted with Amendments up to Nov. 30, 1910. 1*d.* (1*d.*)

STAFF. General. Duties of. (*Von Schellendorff.*) Fourth Edition. 1905. (*Out of print*)

STATIONS OF UNITS OF THE REGULAR FORCES, MILITIA, SPECIAL RESERVE, AND TERRITORIAL FORCE. Quarterly up to No. 45, July 1914. Each 2*d.* (2*d.*) (*Publication suspended*).

STATUTES relating to the War Office and to the Army. 1880. 5*s.* (3*s.* 9*d.*)

STATUTORY POWERS of the Secretary of State, Ordnance Branch. 1879. 5*s.* (3*s.* 9*d.*)

STEAM ENGINES AND BOILERS AND GAS AND OIL ENGINES. Management of. Notes and Memoranda. 1911. 1*d.* (1*d.*)

SUDAN ALMANAC. 1915. Compiled in the Intelligence Department, Cairo. .1*s.* (9*d.*)

SUDAN. BRITISH FORCE IN THE. Standing Orders. 1914. 9*d.* (7*d.*)

SUDAN. The Anglo-Egyptian. A Compendium prepared by Officers of the Sudan Government:—

    Vol. I. Geographical, Descriptive, and Historical (*with Eighty-two Illustrations*). 10*s.* (7*s.* 4*d.*)

    Vol. II. Routes. 7*s.* 6*d.* (5*s.* 5*d.*) (*Not containing Chapter VII., Supplement (A).*)

(As to prices in brackets, see top of page 2.)

SUDAN. The Anglo-Egyptian—*continued.*

> Vol. II. Routes. In Separate Chapters. 1s. (10d.) each:—
> I. and II., *Nil.* III. North-Eastern Sudan. IV. Eastern Sudan.
> V. Central Sudan. VI. South-Eastern Sudan. VII. Bahr-el-
> Ghazal. VIII. Kordofan. IX. North-Western Sudan.
> Ditto. Chapter VII. Supplement (A). Bahr-el-Ghazal. Additional
> Routes. 1s. (10d.)

SUDAN CAMPAIGN. History of the. Two parts, and Maps. 1890. 15s.
(10s. 11d.)

SUPPLY MANUAL (WAR). 1909. 6d. (6d.)

SUPPLY, REORGANIZED SYSTEMS OF, and of Ammunition Supply
of the Expeditionary Force in War, consequent on the Introduction of
Mechanical Transport. Memorandum explaining the. Feb. 1912. 1d. (1d.)

SUPPLY, TRANSPORT, AND BARRACK SERVICES. Regulations.
1908. 9d. (8d.)   *(Under revision)*

SURVEYING. Topographical and Geographical. Text Book of. Second
edition. 1913. 7s. 6d. (5s. 6d.)

> Ditto. 1905. Appendix XI. Tables for the Projection of Graticules for
> squares on 1° side on scale of 1:250,000, and for squares
> on ½° side on scale of 1:125,000; with other Tables used
> in Projecting Maps. 4d. (4d.)
> Ditto. 1905. Appendix XII. Tables for the Projection of Graticules for
> Maps on the scale of 1:1,000,000. 1910. 2d. (2d.)

TACTICAL RIDES AND TOURS ON THE GROUND. The Prepara-
tion and Conduct of. Translated from the German. 1s. 3d. (1s. 1d.)

TELEGRAPHY AND TELEPHONY. Army. Instruction in:—
Vol. I. Instruments. (Reprinted, with Corrections. 1914). 1s. 6d. (1s. 4d.)
Vol. II. Lines. 1909. (Reprinted, with Corrections. 1914). 1s. (11d.)

TELESCOPIC SIGHTS. Handbook. Land Service. 1904. 4d. (4d.)

TERRITORIAL FORCE. (*And see* Equipment; Establishments):—

> Cadet Units in the British Isles. Regulations governing the Formation,
> Organization, and Administration of. 1914. (Reprinted, with Amend-
> ments in Army Orders to Dec. 1, 1914). 1d. (1d.)
> Field Kits. Officers and Men. 1d. (1d.)
> Hospitals, General, of the. Regulations for. 1912. 2d. (2d.)
> Medical Corps. Royal Army. Syllabus of Training. 1914. 1d. (1d.)
> Mobilization of a Territorial Infantry Battalion. (*Reprinted from* THE
> ARMY REVIEW, July 1913.) 3d. (3d.)
> Nursing Service. Standing Orders. 1912. (Reprinted, with Amendments,
> 1914). 1d. (1d.)
> Pay Duties during Embodiment. Instructions in. 2d. (2d.) (*In the press*)
> Regulations for the (including the Territorial Force Reserve), and for
> County Associations. 1912. (Reprinted, with Amendments published
> in Army Orders to Dec. 1, 1914). 6d. (7d.)
> Voluntary Aid:—
> Scheme for the Organization of, in England and Wales. Dec. 1910.
>   (*Out of print*)
>
> > Ditto. Ditto. Amendments. 1d (1d.)
> > Ditto, in Scotland. Oct. 1911. 2d. (2d.)
> > Ditto. Ditto. Amendments. 1d. (1d.)
> > Training. (Extracts from "Medical Corps. Royal Army. Training.
> > 1911,") 6d. (7d.)

(As to prices in brackets, see top of page 2.)

TRACTOR TRIALS held by the Experimental Sub-Committee of the Mechanical Transport Committee at Aldershot, Sept. and Oct. 1903. Report on. **6d.** (5d.)

TRAINING AND MANŒUVRE REGULATIONS. 1913. **4d.** (5d.)

TRANSPORT MANUAL. Field Service. 1905. Part I. Provisional. **4d.** (4d.)

TRANSPORT. MECHANICAL :—
Heavy Pontoon Bridge for use by. Provisional. 1914. **2d.** (2d.)
Regulations for the Appointment of Inspectors of. **1d.** (1d.)

TRANSPORT. PACK. Notes on. **1d.** (1d.)

TRUMPET AND BUGLE SOUNDS for the Army. With Instructions for the Training of Trumpeters and Buglers. 1914. **9d.** (8d.)

TYPHOID (ANTI-) COMMITTEE. Report. 1912. **2s. 6d.** (1s. 11d.)

TYPHOID (ANTI-) INOCULATION COMMITTEE. Report on Blood Changes following Typhoid Inoculation. 1905. **1s. 6d.** (1s. 2d.)

URDU-ENGLISH PRIMER. For the use of Colonial Artillery. 1899. **15s.** (10s. 2d.)

VALISE EQUIPMENT. Instructions for Fitting :—
Pattern 1888 with pattern 1894 Pouch opening outwards. **1895. 1d.** (1d.)
Bandolier pattern. 1903. **2d.** (2d.)

VALPARAISO. The Capture of, in 1891. **1s.** (10d.)

VENEREAL DISEASE. *See* Medical Services.

VETERINARY CORPS. Army :—
Regulations for Admission. 1910. **2d.** (2d.)
Standing Orders. 1906. **4d.** (4d.)

VETERINARY MANUAL (WAR). 1915. **1d.** (1d.)

VETERINARY SERVICES. Army. Regulations. 1906. (Reprinted, with Amendments to Dec. 1, 1914). **3d.** (3d.)

VOLUNTARY AID. *See* Territorial Force.

WAR OFFICE LIST, AND ADMINISTRATIVE DIRECTORY FOR THE BRITISH ARMY. 1914. *Sold by Harrison & Sons.* 45, *Pall Mall.* **5s. net.** *(Under revision)*

WARFARE. *See* Land Warfare.

WATER SUPPLY MANUAL. **1s. 6d.** (1s. 4d.)

WORKS MANUAL. (WAR.) 1913. **4d.** (4d.); Corrections *(In the press)*

X-RAY APPARATUS. Hints regarding the Management and use of. **3d.** (3d.)

YEOMANRY AND MOUNTED RIFLE TRAINING. Parts I. and II. 1912. (Reprinted, with Amendments, 1915). **6d.** (6d.) *(In the press)*

ZULU WAR OF 1879. Narrative of the Field Operations connected with the. 1881. *(Reprinted* 1907.) **3s.** (2s. 4d.)

ND - #0530 - 270225 - C0 - 195/125/3 - PB - 9781908487681 - Matt Lamination